MW01166062

Med-Surg

Medical Surgical
Clinical Nursing Reference

Third Edition

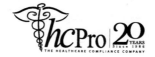

THE HEALTHCARE COMPLIANCE COMPANY

Copyright 2006 HCPro, Inc.

All rights reserved. Printed in the United States of America. 5 4 3 2 1

ISBN: 1-57839-848-7

No part of this publication may be reproduced, in any form or by any means, without prior written consent of HCPro, Inc., or the Copyright Clearance Center (978/750-8400). Please notify us immediately if you have received an unauthorized copy.

HCPro, Inc., provides information resources for the healthcare industry.

Includes references.

Other titles available in the *Quick-E Series:*

- **I.V.** *Intravenous Nursing*
- **E.R.** *Emergency Nursing*
- **Peds** *Pediatric Nursing*
- **O.B.** *Obstetric Nursing*

- **Dysrhythmia**
- **Critical Care**
- **Spanish Guide**
- **Assessment** & *Physical Exam*

Advice given is general. Readers should consult professional counsel for specific legal, ethical, or clinical questions. Arrangements can be made for quantity discounts. For more information, contact:

HCPro, Inc.
P.O. Box 1168
Marblehead, MA 01945
Telephone: 800/650-6787 or 781/639-1872
Fax: 781/639-2982
E-mail: *customerservice@hcpro.com*

Visit HCPro at its World Wide Web sites:
www.hcpro.com and *www.hcmarketplace.com.*

08/2006
20921

Reviewer

Elizabeth R. Santulli,
RN, BSN, MA, COHN-S
Occupational Health Nurse
Washington, DC

This reference work is designed to be used by qualified licensed professionals and/or students under the supervision of a qualified professional. The publisher assumes no responsibilities or liabilities from any effects of the implementation of the information imparted here, nor from any undetected errors or reader misunderstanding of the text. For their protection, readers are urged to practice within their scope as prescribed by the regional professional governing body or the local institution. This work is not intended to supersede or replace any rules, policies, or standards of practice applicable to the user.

Contents

Section Color Code Scheme. **Green:** Lab Values, Units of Measurement, Hormone Guide, Infection Control, Assessment **Blue:** IV Therapy, Nutrition **Red:** BLS, Medications **Gray:** Nursing Diagnoses and References

This book, as others in the *Quick-E Series*, is intended to be used by nurses and nursing students as a quick, portable, and easy-to-use pocket reference. The goal of this volume is not to be exhaustive in its clinical content to the areas of medical-surgical nursing, but rather to provide clinicians with easy access to often-needed information in a clinical setting.

Quick-E: Med-Surg aims to maximize the nurse's time by facilitating information in a durable and portable format ideal for the "bedside" practice. Ultimately, the intent is that this book helps to enhance the quality of patient care through quick access to clinical facts applicable and usable in the medical-surgical practice.

The book is organized by topical content separated by color dividers to facilitate quick location of information. The color dividers are placed throughout the text to help the user thumb through pages and to quickly identify sections and locate material. For the sake of brevity and practicality certain abbreviations and symbols are used throughout the text and assume a basic knowledge of medical terminology by the user. Users are strongly encouraged to adhere to institutional standards in obtaining, interpreting, applying and documenting all clinical findings. Since all individual clinical practice is unique, there is room throughout the text for you to customize this tool with your own clinical notes. Additional information and more in-depth clinical and academic coverage may be found in the "Reference" section.

Happy Nursing!

Laboratory Values*

CBC

RBC	4.7–6.1 million/mm^3 (♂)	**Hgb**	13.5–17.5 g/dl (♂)
	4.2–5.4 million/mm^3 (♀)		12–16 g/dl (♀)
WBC	4300–10800 cells/mm^3	**Hct**	40–54 % (♂)
			37–47 % (♀)
Platelets	150–350 thousand/mm^3	**MCV**	80–94 cu microns
MCH	27–32 pg	**MCHC**	32–36 %

Chemistry

Na	135–148 mEq/L	**K**	3.5–5.0 mEq/L
Cl	98–106 mEq/L	**CO$_2$**	24–32 mEq/L
BUN	7–18 mg/dl	**Uric Acid**	3.0–7.0 mg/dl
Ca	8.5–10.5 mg/dl	**Mg**	1.3–2.1 mEq/L
Creatinine	0.7–1.3 mg/dl (♂)	**Glucose**	
	0.6–1.2 mg/dl (♀)	(fasting)	70–110 mg/dl
Bilirubin		**SGPT** (ALT)	
	Direct 0–0.2 mg/dl		10–55 U/L (♂)
	Total 0.2–1.0 mg/dl		7–30 U/L (♀)
Indirect:	Total minus Direct		
Osmolality	275–295 mOsm/kg	**Anion gap**	8–16 mEg/L
Amylase	50–150 U/L	**Lipase**	4–24 U/L
Alkaline Phosphatase (ALP)		**Lipids**	See page 28
	13–39 U/L (adults)	"Cholesterol Recommendations"	

*Refers to adult values unless otherwise noted

"It's better to be sick than nurse the sick. Sickness is single trouble for the sufferer; but nursing means vexation of the mind, and hard work for the hands besides."

—Euripedes

Sedimentation Rate

Wintrobe 0–9 mm per hour (♂) 0–20 mm per hour (♀)	*Westergren* 1–13 mm per hour (♂) 1–20 mm per hour (♀)

Coagulation

PT	10–14 sec	**PTT**	30–45 sec
APTT	16–25 sec	**ACT**	92–128 sec
FSP	<10 µg/dl	**Platelets**	150-350thousand/mm^3

Cardiac Profile

SGOT (AST)	7–21 U/L (♂) 6–18 U/L (♀)	**SGOT** *with MI* Onset 12–18 hours	Peak 24–48 hours Duration 3–4 days
CK	38–174 U/L (♂) 96–140 U/L (♀)	**CK** *with MI* Onset 4–6 hours	Peak 12–24 hours Duration 3–4 days
CK-MB	0%	**CK-MB** *with MI* Onset 4–6 hours	Peak 12–24 hours Duration 2–3 days
LDH	90–200 U/L	**LDH** *with MI* Onset 24–48 hours	Peak 3–6 days Duration 7–10 days
LDH$_1$ **LDH$_2$**	17.5–28.3% total LDH 30.4–36.4% total LDH	*With MI* $LDH_1 > LDH_2$	Onset 12–24 hours Peak 48 hours Duration Variable
Troponin I At least 1.5µg/ml to 3.1µg/ml for AMI (acute myocardial infarction)		**Myoglobin** References varying for AMI from 50 µg/ml to 120 µg/ml	

Urine Values

Specific Gravity	1.003–1.030	**PH**	4.5–8.0
Osmolality	300–1200 mOsm/L	**Volume**	1200 (600–2500cc/24hrs)
Glucose	Normally not found	**Protein**	Normally not found
Bilirubin	Negative	**Urobilinogen**	Up to 1.0 Ehrlich U

❖ *Consistent appearance of casts and epithelial cells is abnormal.*

Fecal Studies

Occult Blood (FOBT, hemoccult, guaiac)		Negative
Trypsin Positive result is normal	**Ova and Parasites**	Negative

Drug Levels

Digoxin	1–2 ng/ml	**Phenytoin**	10–20 mcg/ml
Theophylline	10–20 mcg/ml	**Barbiturate coma**	10 mg/100ml
Gentamicin	Trough 1–2 mcg/ml Peak 6–8 mcg/ml	**Tobramycin**	Trough 1–2 mcg/ml Peak 6–8 mcg/ml

ABGs

PH	7.35–7.45	**Pao$_2$**	80–100 mm Hg
Paco$_2$	35–45 mm Hg	**HCO$_3$**	22–26 mEq/L
% Sat	95–99	**Base Excess**	±2

Using Lab Values

To assess status:	Consult:
Renal	Urine values, BUN, creatinine, serum electrolytes
Liver	ALP, SGPT, bilirubin (serum and urine), urobilinogen, LDH, PT, cholesterol, hepatitis profile
Pancreatic	Amylase, lipase
Respiratory	ABGs, sputum culture
Cardiac	See *Cardiac Profile*, lipids

Units of Measurement

Temperature

$°F - 32 × 0.5555 = °C$		$°C × 1.8 + 32 = °F$	
°F	**°C**	**°C**	**°F**
0	-17.8	0	32.0
95	35.0	35.0	95.0
96	35.6	35.5	95.9
97	36.1	36.0	96.8
98	36.7	36.5	97.7
99	37.2	37.0	98.6
100	37.8	37.5	99.5
101	38.3	38.0	100.4
102	38.9	38.5	101.3
103	39.4	39.0	102.2
104	40.0	39.5	103.1
105	40.6	40.0	104.0

Weight

$lb/2.2 = Kg$		$Kg × 2.2 = lb$	
lb	**Kg**	**Kg**	**lb**
1	0.5	1	2.2
2	0.9	2	4.4
4	1.8	5	11
10	4.5	10	22
50	22.7	50	110
100	45.5	80	176
150	68.2	90	198
200	90.9	100	220

Equivalents of Measurement

Metric (volume)	Apothecary	Household
1 ml	15 minims	15 drops
15 ml	4 fluidrams	1 tablespoon
30 ml	1 fluid ounce	2 tablespoons
240 ml	8 fluid ounces	1 cup
480 ml (approx. .5 L)	1 pint	1 pint
960 ml (approx. 1 L)	1 quart	1 quart
3840 ml	1 gallon	1 gallon

Hormone Guide

Organ	Hormone	Effect
Adrenal {adrenal cortex}	Mineralocorticoids (mainly aldosterone but over two dozen produced)	↑Na and ↓K; ↑water and BP. *Hyposecretion: Addison's. Hypersecretion: Aldosteronism*
	Glucocorticoids (mainly cortisol)	Blood sugar levels, fat metabolism, protein catabolism, assists body to resist stressors, depress inflamatory and immune responses. *Hyposecretion: Addison's. Hypersecretion: Cushing's*
	Gonadocorticoids (sex hormones, mainly androgens)	Thought to affect ♀ sex drive and provide small amounts of estrogen after menopause
{adrenal medulla}	Epinephrine and noroepinephrine	AKA catecholamines. Sympathetic nervous system. Flight-or-fight. Epi ↑heart and metabolic activities and bronchodilation, noroepi ↑peripheral vasoconstriction.
Gonads (♂ testes, ♀ ovaries)	♀ Estrogen and progesterone	Secondary sex characteristics, maturation of reproductive organs, estrogen promotes uterine changes in menstrual cycle
	♂ Testosterone	Secondary sex characteristics, maturation of reproductive organs, sperm production

"A little rebellion now and then is a good thing."
—Thomas Jefferson

Organ	Hormone	Effect
Pancreas	Glucagon	Hyperglycemic agent. *Persistent low blood sugar levels may be associated with glucagon deficiency*
	Insulin	Lowers blood sugar level and influences protein and fat metabolism. *Hyposecretion: Diabete mellitus. Hyperinsulinism may occur and is commonly from an overdose of insulin*
Parathyroid	Parathyroid hormone	Ca balance. *Surgical removal of gland may result in hypocalcemia, tetany, seizure and death if not corrected*
Pineal	Melatonin	Inhibits gonadotropic functions, sleep/wake cycle
Pituitary	Growth hormone	Body growth, protein and fat metabolism. *Hyposecretion: Pituitary dwarfism. Hypersecretion: giantism (children), acromegaly (adults).*
	Thyroid stimulating hormone (TSH)	Growth and maintenance of thyroid gland
	Adrenocorticotropic hormone (ACTH)	Growth and maintenance of adrenal cortex
	Prolactin	Milk secretion, maintenance of corpus luteum
	Follicle stimulating hormone (FSH) and luteinizing hormone (LH), referred to as gonadotropins	Regulate function of gonads (both ♂ and ♀)

Organ	Hormone	Effect
Pituitary (cont.)	Oxytocin	Uterine contraction and ejection of milk
	Antidiuretic hormone (ADH)	Inhibits urine formation. *Hyposecretion: Diabetes insipidus, most commonly from hypothalmic trauma*
Thymus	Thymopoietin, thymosin	Primary central gland of the lymphatic system. T cells develop here, essential for development of normal immune response
Thyroid *(goiter: enlarged thyroid gland)*	Thyroxine T_4, triiodothyronine T_3	↑Rate of cellular metabolism in body (BMR). Affects virtually every cell in the body, regulates tissue growth and development, nervous system development and reproductive capabilities. Plays a role in BP maintenance and temperature regulation. *Hyposecretion: Myxedema (in children, severe hypothyrodism: Cretinism). Hypersecretion: Grave's.*
	Calcitonin	Antagonist of parathyroid hormone, ↓blood Ca levels

"I have always held firmly to the thought that each one of us can do a little to bring some portion of misery to an end."
—Albert Schweitzer

Organ	Hormone	Effect
Other	Prostaglandins (associated with plasma membrane)	Mediate hormone responses, stimulates smooth muscles of arterioles or uterus, ↑HCl and pepsin secretion by stomach, ↑inflamation and pain, induce fever
	Gastrin (stomach), enterogastrin, secretin, cholecystokinin (duodenum)	Regulate secretion of HCl, bicarbonate, and digestive enzymes
	Erythropoietin (kidney)	Act on bone marrow to ↑RBC production
	Atrial natriuretic factor (atrium of heart)	↓BP

First Line of Defense: The Immune System

Neutrophilis:	Defense against bacteria
Eosinophils:	Allergic reactions
Basophils:	Homeostasis in microvascular
B-Lymphocytes:	Active immunity
T-Lymphocytes:	Protects foreign cells
Monocytes:	Phagocytes

"There never was a good war or a bad peace."
—Benjamin Franklin

Infection Control

Standard Precautions

- The CDC defines standard precautions as a set of precautions designed to prevent transmission of human immunodeficiency virus (HIV), hepatitis B virus (HBV), hepatitis C virus (HCV), and other bloodborne pathogens, and designed to reduce the risk of transmission of pathogens from moist body substances. "Standard precautions are designed to reduce the risk of transmission of microorganisms from both recognized and unrecognized sources of infection in hospitals."*

- All patients are potential sources of infectious diseases.

- Gloves are considered the minimal barrier. Gloves will not protect you from injury by sharp objects. Gloves should always be changed after contact with patient, and hands should be washed immediately after removal of gloves.

- If the generation of droplets, or splashing of blood or body fluids, is anticipated during therapy/procedure, additional protective barriers should be worn (gowns, masks, goggles).

- Dispose of blood-contaminated items properly and, again, assume that they are potentially infectious.

- Utilize needleless, or safety-engineered products in accordance with manufacturer's instructions and facility policy.

- Dispose of sharps properly and carefully (to prevent breakage of materials and injury, do not over-stuff containers; follow manufacturer's instructions for filling limits and correct handling).

- Follow product instructions to maintain product sterility. Maintain aseptic technique with infusion procedures. Remember: *hand washing is the primary infection control measure.*

* Center for Disease Control and Prevention. 1996. Guideline for isolation precautions in hospitals. *www.cdc.gov/ncidod/dhqp/gl_isolation_standard.html*

Bloodborne Pathogens: Occupational Exposure

• **Hepatitis B (HBV)** Transmitted by percutaneous or mucosal exposure to blood and serum derived body fluids from infected individuals. Vaccine is available and recommended. Vaccine should be offered to exposed, unvaccinated person and, if exposure source is known to be positive, hepatitis B immune globulin (HBIG) should be given as treatment (tx), preferably within 24 hours of exposure. Risk of infection for unvaccinated person: 6–30%.

• **Hepatitis C (HCV)** Most common chronic bloodborne infection in the United States. Most individuals are chronically infected and do not know about it, since they show no clinical signs or symptoms. Virus is transmitted primarily through large or repeated direct percutaneous exposures to blood. Immune globulin and antiviral agents (e.g., interferon with or without ribavirin) are not recommended for post-exposure prophylaxes of hepatitis C. No vaccine is available. Risk of infection approximately 1.8% for needle stick or cut (risk from a blood splash unknown but believed to be small).

• **Human Immunodeficiency Virus (HIV)** As of printing, no vaccine is available although many are currently being researched. Prophylactic tx is not recommended for all occupational exposures to HIV because most exposures do not lead to infection, and the tx drugs may have serious side effects. Decision for tx should be made in consultation with healthcare provider. Current tx recommendations include a basic 4-week regimen of two drugs (zidovudine [ZDV] and lamivudine [3TC]; 3TC and stavudine [d4T]; or didanosine [ddI] and d4T) for most HIV exposures and an expanded regimen that includes the addition of a third drug for HIV exposures that pose an increased risk for transmission. Recommendations are guidelines and may be modified clinically as needed. Risk of infection from needle stick or cut is 0.3%. Risk after exposure of the eye, nose, or mouth to HIV infected blood is 0.1%. Risk after exposure of the skin to HIV infected blood is <0.1%.

Assessment

Abdominopelvic Quadrants

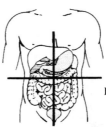

Right Upper Quadrant
Liver
Gallbladder
Pylorus
Head of pancreas
Duodenum
Upper right kidney

Left Upper Quadrant
Left lobe of liver
Spleen
Stomach
Body of pancreas
Left kidney

Right Lower Quadrant
Lower right kidney
Cecum
Appendix
Ascending colon
R fallopian tube (♀)
R ovary (♀)
R ureter, Bladder (dis-
tended)

Left Lower Quadrant
Descending colon
Sigmoid colon
L ureter
Bladder (distended)
L fallopian tube (♀)
L ovary (♀)

Assessment Scales

Pitting Edema		Pulse	
+1	5mm depth	0	Absent
+2	8-10 mm depth	+1	Decreased, thready
+3	> 10 mm depth, up to 30 sec	+2	Normal
+4	>20 mm depth, longer than 30 sec	+3	Full, bounding
Deep Tendon Reflexes		**Muscle Movement of Extremities**	
0	Absent	0	No contraction
1+	Diminished	1	Slight contraction
2+	Normal	2	Active with gravity eliminated
3+	Increased	3	Active with gravity
4+	Hyperactive, clonus	4	Active, some resistance
		5	Full strength against resistance

Cranial Nerves

Cranial Nerve	Type	Function	Assessment
I Olfactory	Sensory	Smell	Test with non-noxious smells such as orange, coffee, soap, or vanilla.
II Optic	Sensory	Vision	Visual acuity.
III Oculomotor	Mixed	Ocular movement, pupil constriction, lens shape, eyelids	Check pupils for size, light reaction and accommodation. Assess extraocular movements.
IV Trochlear	Motor	Eye movement	
V Trigeminal	Mixed	Chewing, sensation of face, cornea, scalp, mouth and nose	Palpate chewing muscles as client clenches teeth. Check for sensation on face.
VI Abducens	Motor	Lateral eye movement	*
VII Facial	Mixed	Taste on anterior tongue, facial muscles, close eye, saliva, tears	Lift eyebrows, smile. Identify taste of safe substance (lemon, salt).
VIII Acoustic	Sensory	Hearing and balance	Hearing acuity.
IX Glossopharyngeal	Mixed	Gag reflex, taste on posterior tongue, swallowing, parotid gland, carotid reflex	Assess uvula and soft palate placement with tongue depress while client says "ahh." Uvula to midline. Note gag reflex.
X Vagus	Mixed	Talking and swallowing, general carotid sensation, sinus, and reflex	
XI Spinal	Motor	Trapezius and sternomastoid movement	Shrug shoulders. Rotate head to side against resistance.
XII Hypoglossal	Motor	Tongue movement	Note speech. Midline forward thrust of tongue.

* Assessed together with cranial nerves III and IV

Neurologic Reference

Sign	Description
Babinski	Sole of foot is stroked. Abnormal: Dorsiflexion of big toe and fanning of the toes. Upper motor neuron dysfunction. Normal: Plantar flexion.
Brudzinski	Passive neck flexion trigger flexion of the hip and knee. Pathologic reflex indicating meningeal irritation.
Kernig	Resistance to full extension of the leg at the knee when the hip is flexed. Pathologic reflex indicating meningeal irritation.
Oculocephalic (doll's eye maneuver)	Head rotated from side to side. Abnormal: Eyes move with the head fixed in place. This is a normal response in newborns but disappears as ocular fixation develops. Indicates brainstem injury. Normal: Eyes remain in the initial position, then turn slowly in the direction of head rotation.
Oculovestibular (ice water calorics, also called Barany's test)	Ear alternately irrigated with hot and cold water. Abnormal: *Supratentorial or metabolic lesion*, eyes move slowly toward irrigated ear and remain there for 2–3 minutes. Absent fast return to midline. *Brainstem lesion*, downward deviation and rotary jerking of one eye. *Severe brainstem injury*, no response. Normal: Hot water irrigation produces a rotatory nystagmus towards irrigated ear. Cold water produces a rotatory nystagmus away from irrigated ear
Decorticate	Flexion of upper extremities, legs may be extended. Indicates lesion to the mesencephalic region of the brain
Decerebrate	Extension of upper extremities with internal rotation, legs may be extended. Indicates brainstem lesion

• **Spinal Cord** 31 Pairs of spinal nerves originate from the cord: 8 cervical, 12 thoracic, 5 lumbar, 5 sacral, 1 coccygeal. Lesions below first thoracic vertebra may produce *paraplegia*. Lesions above first thoracic vertebra may produce *quadriplegia*. Lesions that completely transect the spinal cord cause loss of motor and sensory function below the level of injury.

🖤 **Dysreflexia** state in which an individual with a spinal cord injury at T7 or above experiences a life threatening uninhibited sympathetic response of the nervous system to a noxious stimulus. S+S include pallor below the injury, red splotches on skin above the injury, paroxysmal hypertension (sudden periodic ↑BP systolic >140 and diastolic >90mm Hg), headache, blurred vision, chest pain, horner's syndrome, metallic taste in mouth, gooseflesh formation when skin is cooled. Treatment: Elevate head, identify and remove noxious stimulus (bladder or bowel distention, skin irritation etc), monitor BP closely, have available antihypertensives as physician prescribes.

Breath Sounds

❖ Auscultate in a systematic manner both anterior and posterior chest walls starting from the apices and working from side to side, downward to bases. Do not auscultate over bone or breast tissue.

Common Causes of Apnea: Airway Obstruction

• Asthma	• Pneumothorax/Hemothorax	• Obstructive Sleep Apnea
• Bronchospasm	• Mucus Plug	• Secretion retention
• Chronic bronchitis	• Obstruction by tongue or	• Tracheal or bronchial
• Foreign body aspiration	tumor	rupture

Adventitious Sounds

Crackles	Air that contains serous secretions. Bubbling, wet sound (a.k.a. rales). Pneumonia, CHF, bronchitis, emphysema.
Wheezes	Air flowing through narrow airways. High pitch, musical quality. Acute asthma, bronchitis.
Stridor	High pitch, crowing sound. Croup, airway obstruction, acute epiglotitis (children).
Rub	Coarse and low pitch. Pleuritis.

Assess

Pitch	Is it high or low?
Timing	When is it occurring? Late or early? Inspiratory or expiratory?
Quality	Is it loud or soft? Coarse or fine? Is it continuous or intermittent?
Location	Where on the chest wall was sound auscultated?

Chest Tube Drainage

Water Seal Chamber	Collection Chamber	Suction Chamber
Usual level at 2–3 cm. Bubbling indicates air leak in system. If bubbling, clamp near client. If bubbling stops, leak within client or at insertion site. Notify physician. If bubbling does not stop, leak is in the system. Locate leak by clamping along tubing. Replace and retape equipment prn.	If drainage >100 ml/hr for 2 hours or sudden change in amount of bloody drainage, notify physician. If drainage is decreased, check for kinks and clots. Consult your local protocol in regards to milking tube.	Usual 15-25 cm water. Maintain constant, gentle bubbling. Maintain appropriate fluid level. ❧ Keep a bottle of sterile water and sterile petroleum gauze available. If system interrupted, tube should be placed in a few cms of sterile water while system reestablished. Gauze for applying to chest wall if tube is accidentally removed.

Oxygen Delivery Systems

Nasal Cannula	4–6 L/min deliver 35-40% FIo_2. Higher flow rates dry airway mucosa and not recommended.
Simple Mask	Minimum flow of 5-6 L/min. 10-12 L/min deliver 55–65% FIo_2.
Nonrebreathing Mask	Attached reservoir allows theoretical delivery of 90–100% FIo_2. In practice, usually delivers up to 70% FIo_2 at 10 L/min.
Venturi Mask	Delivers controlled FIo_2 at specific rates. 4 L/min (24%), 6 L/min (28%), 8 L/min (35%), and 10 L/min (40% Flo_2).

Cardiac Assessment

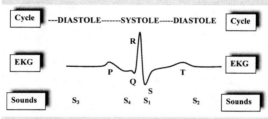

Cycle	---DIASTOLE------SYSTOLE-----DIASTOLE	Cycle
EKG		EKG
Sounds	S_3 S_4 S_1 S_2	Sounds

Murmur Scale

Grade	Description
I	Barely audible
II	Audible
III	Moderately loud, no thrill
IV	Loud, no thrill
V	Very loud, associated with a thrill
VI	Very loud, thrill, audible with Stethoscope off the chest

Heart Sounds

S_1	Beginning systole. Loudest at apex. Caused by closure of AV valves.
S_2	Loudest at base. Caused by closure of semilunar valves.
S_3	May be normal when in children and young adults. Associated with CHF. Abnormal over age 35 termed *ventricular gallop*.
S_4	May occur in adults >40 without disease. Pathologic S_4 termed *atrial gallop*.

Auscultatory Areas

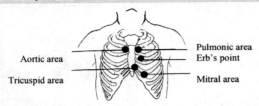

Aortic area

Tricuspid area

Pulmonic area

Erb's point

Mitral area

• Erbs's point is frequently the area to which aortic or pulmonic sounds radiate. Valve areas are not over actual anatomic sites but are where sounds produced by the valves are best heard.

Pacemaker Terminology

Fixed-rate *(asynchronous)* Paces at fixed rate regardless of spontaneous cardiac activity.

Demand *(synchronous)* Paces only when heart's intrinsic pacemaker fails to function at a predetermined rate.

AV Sequential *(dual-chamber pacing)* Paces both atrium and ventricle in sequence.

Pacemaker Codes

Code	Description	Code	Description
AOO	Atrial (A) fixed rate, no sensing	AAT	A demand, paced/sensed, triggered response to sensing
VOO	Ventricular (V) fixed rate, no sensing	VAT	AV synchronous, V pacing, A sensing, triggered response
DOO	AV sequential fixed, no sensing	DVI	AV sequential, A+V pacing, V sensing, inhibited response
VVI	V demand, V paced/sensed, inhibited response to sensing	VDD	A synchronous, V inhibited, V pacing, A+V sensing, inhibited response to sensing in V and triggered response to sensing in A
VVT	V demand, V paced/sensed, triggered response to sensing		
AAI	A demand, paced/sensed, inhibited response to sensing	DDD	Universal, A+V senses and paced inhibited in V, triggered in A

Bowel Sounds

Normal	5–3 times per minute
Hyperactive	Loud, high pitch, rushing, tinkling sounds. Borborygmus (stomach growling), signal increased motility. Occur with early mechanical bowel obstruction (high pitched), gastroenteritis, brisk diarrhea, laxative use, subsiding paralytic ileus.
Hypoactive	Signal decreased motility due to inflammation. Occur with peritonitis, paralytic ileus as following abdominal surgery, and late bowel obstruction. Also occurs with pneumonia and electrolyte imbalance. A "silent" abdomen is uncommon. Listen for 5 minutes before deciding that bowel sounds are completely absent.

Pressure Sore Scale

Stage I	Non-blanchable erythema of intact skin; indicates likely progression to ulceration.
Stage II	Partial thickness skin loss; involves epidermis and/or dermis. This superficial ulcer appears as an abrasion, blister, or shallow crater.
Stage III	Full-thickness skin loss; involves subcutaneous tissue and may extend down to (but excludes) the fascia. This deeper ulcer appears as a deep crater and may have undermining of adjacent tissues.
Stage IV	Full-thickness skin loss with destruction of tissue including the muscle, bone, or supporting structures. Undermining of adjacent structures may be present.

*Wounds covered with eschar may not be staged unless the eschar is removed to determine the extent of underlying tissue destruction/necrosis. Never "de-stage" a pressure sore as it heals, i.e., a Stage III sore later becomes a "healing Stage III sore" *not* a Stage II or Stage I sore.

Quick-E Head-To-Toe 5-Minute Assessment

- Gather and review hx and meds from chart, kardex, or report.
- General appearance (loc, gait, mood, affect, speech, hearing, *how are you feeling, what is bothering you?*).
- Head and neck (eye contact, pupils, skin condition, scalp, lips and tongue, cervical lymph nodes, neck vessels, *trouble swallowing, poor appetite, drinking O.K.?*).
  - Pupillary assessment size:
    - Pinpoint
    - Small
    - Moderate
    - Large
    - Dilated
- Upper extremities (patent pulses bilaterally, skin temp and turgor, grasp, ROM, *any pain or trouble moving?*).
- Anterior and posterior chest wall (inspect, palpate and auscultate). Listen for extra heart sounds, murmurs.
  - Heart Sounds
    - *Normal:* S1
                 S2
    - *Abnormal:* S3—lub DUB dub
                   S4—lub dub DUB
- Abdomen (first inspect, then auscultate, then palpate). Note bowel sounds, presence of abdominal rigidity or enlarged organs. Light palpation first followed by deeper palpation, *any pain, are bowels moving fine, are you voiding O.K.?*
- Lower extremities (patent pulses bilaterally, skin temp and turgor, capillary refill, assess strength by asking to push ball of foot against your hand, ROM, note any edema, *any problems moving, any calf tenderness?*).

Quick-E Head-To-Toe 5-Minute Assessment (cont.)

Normal Blood Pressure

	Top (systolic)	Bottom (diastolic)
Optimal	less than 120	less than 80
Normal	less than 130	less than 85
High normal	130–139	85–90
Hypertensive	140 or greater	90 or greater

Italics are questions for client. Refer to other portions of the book for specific techniques.

> "Any sufficiently advanced technology
> is indistinguishable from magic."
> —Arthur C. Clarke

Intravenous Therapy

Site Assessment

Color	Redness, blanching, translucence, discoloration
Look for	Hematoma, bruising, swelling, streak formation, leakage, bleeding, purulent drainage, tissue necrosis.
Feel for	Cording, skin tightness, pitting, induration. Assess for presence of pain, numbness and circulatory impairment (capillary refill, pulse).

Infiltration Scale

Value	Interpretation
0	No clinical symptoms
1	Skin blanched. *Edema < 1 inch.* Cool to touch. With or without pain.
2	Skin blanched. *Edema 1–6 inches.* Cool to touch. With our without pain.
3	Skin blanched, *translucent. Gross edema > 6 inches.* Cool to touch. *Mild-moderate pain. Possible numbness.*
4	Skin blanched, translucent. Skin tight, leaking, discolored, bruised, swollen. Gross edema > 6 inches. *Deep pitting tissue edema. Circulatory impairment. Moderate-severe pain. Infiltration of any amount of blood product, irritant, or vesicant.*

Phlebitis Scale

Value	Interpretation
0	No clinical symptoms.
1+	Redness with or without pain. Edema may or may not be present. No streak, no palpable cord.
2+	Redness with or without pain. Edema may or may not be present. Streak formation, no palpable cord.
3+	Redness with or without pain. Edema may or may not be present. Streak formation, palpable cord.

Catheter Gauge Selection

- Catheter gauge selection depends on clinical factors such as prescribed therapy, diagnosis, medical history, activity level, age, and status of veins.
- Use the shortest length and smallest diameter catheter that will get the job done. Remember, *the smaller the catheter gauge number, the larger the diameter*. General considerations as follows: *

Gauge	Uses	Implications
16	Large fluid/volume; rapid infusions (high-risk surgical procedures, trauma).	↑ Likelihood of pain on insertion (? anesthesia). Large vein needed. ↑ likelihood of irritation to vein wall.
18	Surgery, viscous solutions (whole blood, packed RBCs). Various emergent situations.	Large vein needed to accommodate catheter.
20	Routine infusions and routine IV access. Minor surgical procedures.	Frequently selected gauge size.
22	Suitable for most infusions at slower rates. Recommended for small and/or fragile veins. Not appropriate for rapid flow rates.	Easier to insert into small, thin, fragile veins, but may be difficult to insert into tough skin.
24, 26	Slower flow rates. Neonatal, pediatric, and elderly patients.	Easier to insert into extremely small veins; difficult to insert into tough skin.

*Consult local institutional policies for specific guidelines and protocols as applicable

Tonicity and Fluids

- **Isotonic:** Approximately same tonicity as blood plasma. Generally used for volume replacement and maintenance (D_5W, 0.9% saline).
- **Hypotonic:** These solutions contain fewer particles than the solution inside the cell. Used for free water replacement (0.45% saline, Isolyte, Normosol).
- **Hypertonic:** Solutions that contain a greater concentration of particles than that the cell. Used to draw excess fluid from cells and interstitial spaces (mannitol).
- **Crystalloids:** Balanced salt solutions used for both maintenance and replacement therapy (0.9% saline, Lactated Ringer's, D_5W).
- **Colloids:** Salt solutions containing oncotically active particles. Generally used in later stages of loss to help maintain hemodynamic stability and supplement volume (Plasmanate, Hetastarch, Dextran).

❖ Approximate adult fluid intake 50ml/kg/day. 1 liter of fluid = 1kg (2.2lb).

Feeding Tubes

- **Jejunal tubes** ("J" tubes): Various kinds according to how inserted. They include needle catheter jejunostomy (NCJ), percutaneous endoscopic jejunal (PEJ), and nasojejunal tubes. Usually for long-term nutritional maintenance and clients with high risk for aspiration. Verify tube placement according to institutional policy. Standard methods include aspiration of stomach contents (except for NCJ), use of external graduation marks (nasojejunal), and X-ray.

- **Gastrotomy tubes** ("G" tubes): Include percutaneous endoscopic gastric (PEG), surgical, balloon, and low profile gastrostomy tubes. Verify tube placement according to institutional policy. Standard methods include use of external graduation marks, aspiration of stomach contents (in a low profile gastrostomy tube, open the anti-reflux valve first), air auscultation, and X-ray.

- **Nasogastric tubes** ("NG" tubes): Usually temporary, also used to aspirate stomach contents and decompress stomach. Tube placememt: Measure from bridge of nose to ear lobe to xiphoid process, note marking. Verify tube placement according to institutional policy. Standard methods include aspiration of stomach contents, air auscultation, and X-ray.

❖ If in doubt about stomach contents, check pH of aspirate:
  gastric pH 1.0–3.5.

"Work is accomplished by those employees
who have not yet reached their level of incompetence."
—Laurence J. Peter, *The Peter Principle*

Feeding Tube Complications and Management

Complication	Contributing factor	Management
Pulmonary aspiration	Tube in respiratory tract. Regurgitation of feeding.	Verify placement prior to feeding. Add food coloring to formula to facilitate diagnosis. ↑HOB 300 during feedings. Keep ET or trache cuff inflated if possible. Ensure proper gastric emptying (aspirate prior to feeding. Generally volumes >150ml or 110-120% of hourly rate considered excessive).
Diarrhea	Meds, malnutrition, hypertonic formulas or meds, contaminated formula.	Evaluate meds. Consult physician about diluting, slowing feedings, or using continuous feedings. Discard feeding containers and sets q24hr, hang formula no more than 4-8 hr unless prepackaged in sterile set. Keep open formula containers refrigerated and discard within 24hr.
Constipation	Low residue formula. Low fluid intake.	Consult physician about using fiber containing formulas. If no fluid restriction, ensure fluid intake is 50ml/kg/day.
Gastric retention	Neural impairment or serious illness/trauma.	Measure residuals q4-6hr or before feeding. Consult physician about use of "J tube." Consult physician about use of Reglan to stimulate gastric emptying. Encourage client to lie on right side unless contraindicated.
Tube occlusion	Sedimentation of formula or meds.	Avoid use of crushed tablets. Consult pharmacist about elixirs or suspensions. Irrigate tube with water before and after meds and feedings. Continuous feeding, irrigate q4-8hr. Use of soda or cranberry juice has been shown to coagulate whole protein tube feeding formula and may perpetuate the clog. Use of meat tenderizer is uncertain since they are not activated unless heated to high temps. Never insert a device (stylet or guidewire) into a feeding tube for unclogging. Consult physician about use of a pancreatic enzyme solution (Viokase).

Recommended Dietary Daily Allowances (RDAs)

Age (Yrs)	Energy (kcal)	Protein (g)	Vit A (µg RE)	Vit D (µg)	Vit E (mg α-TE)	Vit K (µg)	Vit C (mg)	Thiamin (mg)	Riboflavin (mg)	Niacin (mg NE)	Vitamin B6 (mg)	Folate (µg)	Vit B12 (µg)	Calcium (mg)	Phosphorus (mg)	Magnesium (mg)	Iron (mg)	Zinc (mg)	Iodine (µg)	Selenium (µg)
Males																				
11-14	2500	45	1000	10	10	45	50	1.3	1.5	17	1.7	150	2.0	1200	1200	270	12	15	150	40
15-18	3000	59	1000	10	10	65	60	1.5	1.8	20	2.0	200	2.0	1200	1200	400	12	15	150	50
19-24	2900	58	1000	10	10	70	60	1.5	1.7	19	2.0	200	2.0	1200	1200	350	10	15	150	70
25-50	2900	63	1000	5	10	80	60	1.5	1.7	19	2.0	200	2.0	800	800	350	10	15	150	70
51+	2300	63	1000	5	10	80	60	1.2	1.4	15	2.0	200	2.0	800	800	350	10	15	150	70
Females																				
11-14	2200	46	800	10	8	45	50	1.1	1.3	15	1.4	150	2.0	1200	1200	280	15	12	150	45
15-18	2200	44	800	10	8	55	60	1.1	1.3	15	1.5	180	2.0	1200	1200	300	15	12	150	50
19-24	2200	46	800	10	8	60	60	1.1	1.3	15	1.6	180	2.0	1200	1200	280	15	12	150	55
25-50	2200	50	800	5	8	65	60	1.1	1.3	15	1.6	180	2.0	800	800	280	15	12	150	55
51+	1900	50	800	5	8	65	60	1.0	1.2	13	1.6	180	2.0	800	800	280	10	12	150	55
Pregnant	+300	60	800	10	10	65	70	1.5	1.6	17	2.2	400	2.2	1200	1200	320	30	15	175	65
Lactating																				
1st 6 mo.	+500	65	1300	10	12	65	95	1.6	1.8	20	2.1	280	2.6	1200	1200	355	15	19	200	75
2nd 6 mo.	+500	62	1200	10	11	65	90	1.6	1.7	20	2.1	260	2.6	1200	1200	340	15	16	200	75

Determing Body Mass Index (BMI)

BMI (kg/m²)	19	20	21	22	23	24	25	26	27	28	29	30	35	40
Height (in)	Weight (lb)													
58	91	96	100	105	110	115	119	124	129	134	138	143	167	191
59	94	99	104	109	114	119	124	128	133	138	143	148	173	198
60	97	102	107	112	118	123	128	133	138	143	148	153	179	204
61	100	106	111	116	122	127	132	137	143	148	153	158	185	211
62	104	109	115	120	126	131	136	142	147	153	158	164	191	218
63	107	113	118	124	130	135	141	146	152	158	163	169	197	225
64	110	116	122	128	134	140	145	151	157	163	169	174	204	232
65	114	120	126	132	138	144	150	156	162	168	174	180	210	240
66	118	124	130	136	142	148	155	161	167	173	179	186	216	247
67	121	127	134	140	146	153	159	166	172	178	185	191	223	255
68	125	131	138	144	151	158	164	171	177	184	190	197	230	262
69	128	135	142	149	155	162	169	176	182	189	196	203	236	270
70	132	139	146	153	160	167	174	181	188	195	202	207	243	278
71	136	143	150	157	165	172	179	186	193	200	208	215	250	286
72	140	147	154	162	169	177	184	191	199	206	213	221	258	294
73	144	151	159	166	174	182	189	197	204	212	219	227	265	302
74	148	155	163	171	179	186	194	202	210	218	225	233	272	311
75	152	160	168	176	184	192	200	208	216	224	232	240	279	319
76	156	164	172	180	189	197	205	213	221	230	238	246	287	328

Locate the patient's weight in pounds in the row to the right of his/her height in inches. The corresponding figure at the top is the patient's BMI. A BMI of 30 or greater indicates increased risk associated with weight. For persons with added risk factors, a BMI of 27 or more indicates increased risk.

Estimating Ideal Body Weight (IBW) by Gender/Height

Males		Females	
Height	**Weight Allowance***	**Height**	**Weight Allowance***
First 5 feet of height	106#	First 5 feet of height	100#
Each added inch	Add 6#	Each added inch	Add 5#
Example: Male 5'10"	IBW = 166#	Example: Female 5'4"	IBW = 120#

*10% ± allowance based on build

Relative Health Risk by BMI and Waist Size

BMI	Waist < 40 inches (♂), 35 inches (♀)	Waist > 40 inches (♂), 35 inches (♀)
<18.5		
18.5-24.9		
25.0-29.9	Increased	High
30-34.9	High	Very High
35-39.9	Very High	Very High
≥ 40	Extremely High	Extremely High

Vitamins: Source and Action

Vitamin	Function	Source	Deficiency
A (retinol)	Production of rhodopsin (visual purple).	Liver, cream, butter, whole milk, egg yolk, green and yellow vegetables, yellow fruits	Xerophthalmia
Provitamin A (carotene)	Formation and maintenance of epitheleal tissue. Toxic in large amounts.		Night blindness, skin and mucous membrane infections, faulty tooth formation
D	Absorption of Calcium and phosphorus. Toxic in large amounts.	Fish oils, fortified milk	Rickets, faulty bone growth, osteomalacia in adults
E	Antioxidant with Vitamin A and unsaturated fatty acids. Hemopoiesis, reproduction.	Vegetable oils	Hemolysis of RBCs, possible protection of unsaturated fatty acids
K	Blood clotting. Toxic in large amounts.	Green leafy vegetables, cheese, egg yolk, liver	Bleeding tendencies, poor coagulation
C	Collagen and fibrous tissue formation, aids in fighting bacterial infections.	Citrus fruits, tomatoes, green leafy vegetables	Scurvy, bruising, megaloblastic anemia
Thiamin B_1	Carbohydrate metabolism.	Pork, beef, liver, whole grains, legumes	Beriberi
Riboflavin B_2	Nutrient metabolism, prevents cataracts.	Milk, liver, cheese, eggs, green leafy vegetables	Cheilosis, local inflammation, desquamation, glossitis

Vitamins: Source and Action (cont.)

Vitamin	Function	Source	Deficiency
Niacin	Involved in ATP metabolism.	Meat, peanuts, enriched grains	Pellagra
Pyridoxine B_6	Amino acid metabolism.	Wheat, corn, meat, liver	Hypochromic microcytic anemia
Folic Acid B_9	Essential for cell growth and reproduction.	Spinach and other green leafy vegetables, liver, lima beans, nuts	Poor growth; graying hair; glossitis, stomatitis; need for folic acid increased in pregnacy, infancy, and by stress
Cobalamin B_{12}	Coenzyme in protein synthesis.	Liver, meat, eggs, cheese	Extrinsic factor in pernicious anemia

Cholesterol Recommendations (Lipids)

LDL Cholesterol		Triglycerides	
<100	Optimal	<150 mg/dL	Normal
100–129	Near optimal/above optimal	150–199 mg/dL	Borderline-high
130–159	Borderline high	200–499 mg/dL	High
160–189	High	500 mg/dL	Very high
190	Very high		
Total Cholesterol		**HDL Cholesterol**	
<200	Desirable	<40	Low
200–239	Borderline high	60	High
240	High		

"We boil at different degrees."
—Ralph Waldo Emerson

Cardiopulmonary Resuscitation (CPR)

- Determine if unresponsive.
- Activate EMS (call 911), get automated external defibrillator (AED).[1]
- Open airway, check for breathing (look, listen, and feel).[2]
- If not breathing, give 2 slow breaths[3] and check circulation (pulse).[4]
- If breaths not successful, reposition and reattempt. If unsuccessful, treat for airway obstruction if necessary.[3]
- If no pulse, begin compressions (see chart on p. 31) until AED arrives.
- *AED not recommended in infants/children <8 years old* (approx. 25kg body weight). AED use in children ≥ 8 is a Class IIb recommendation (fair to good).
- All rescuers should "push hard and push fast." Compression of the chest should be at a rate of 100 compressions per minute for all victims (except newborns).
- 30:2 compression-to-ventilation ratio for all victims with 1-rescuer CPR.
- 15:2 compression-to-ventilation ratio for 2-rescuer CPR for infants and children.
- Reassess after 5 compression/ventilation cycles (2 minutes of CPR) by checking pulse.
- If no pulse/no signs of circulation, continue CPR.
- If signs of circulation are present, check breathing. If inadequate breathing, continue rescue breathing, 1 breath every 5 seconds.
- If breathing is adequate, place in a recovery position and monitor.

See *CPR Notes* on the following page.

Basic Life Support Notes

1. Getting Help

Generally, three actions must occur at once at the scene of a cardiac arrest: Activation of EMS (or resuscitation team in a hospital), CPR, and use of AED. When two or more rescuers are present, these actions can be initiated simultaneously (see *Automated External Defibrillator* Section on pages 32–33 for AED use).

"Phone first" to activate EMS as soon as emergency is recognized. If victim is <8 years old, then "phone fast" (begin CPR for approximately 1 minute then activate EMS). Exceptions include:

      1. Near-drowning, "phone fast," all ages
      2. Arrest associated with trauma, "phone fast," all ages
      3. Drug overdoses, "phone fast," all ages
      4. Cardiac arrest in children known to be at high risk for
         arrhythmias, "phone first," all ages

2. Airway

Use the "head tilt-chin lift" technique. Use the "jaw-thrust" technique if there is a suspected spine injury.

3. Breathing

Deliver mouth-to-mouth or mouth-to-mask rescue breaths—two breaths at 1 second/breath—to reduce risk of gastric inflation. If unable to ventilate, reposition, reopen airway, and attempt to ventilate again. If still unable to ventilate, consider foreign body airway obstruction: Perform Heimlich maneuver (abdominal thrusts) up to 5 times, open the airway using the "tongue-jaw lift," perform a finger sweep to remove foreign object, and attempt to ventilate. Repeat until obstruction is cleared or other procedures are available to establish a patent airway. The finger sweep is to be used only on the unresponsive-unconscious adult with a complete foreign body airway obstruction. For child and infant victims: look in mouth, if no foreign bodies are visible, do not perform finger sweep. If foreign bodies are visible, you may remove them.

4. Circulation

Signs of circulation include normal breathing, coughing, or movement. Pulse check should take no more than 10 seconds.

2005 Updates for BLS/HCP* ABCD Maneuvers for Infants, Children, and Adults (Newborn/Neonatal Information Not Included)

MANEUVER	ADULT Lay rescuers ≥ 8years HCP: Adolescent or older	CHILD Lay rescuers: 1 to 8 years HCP: 1 year to adolescent	INFANT Under 1 year
ACTIVATE Emergency Response Number (1- rescuer)	Activate when victim found unresponsive. **HCP**: if asphyxial arrest likely, call after 5 cycles (2 minutes) of CPR.	Activate after performing 5 cycles of CPR. For sudden, witnessed collapse, activate after verifying that victim unresponsive.	Activate after performing 5 cycles of CPR. For sudden, witnessed collapse, activate after verifying that victim unresponsive.
AIRWAY	Head tilt-chin lift (HCP: suspected trauma, use jaw thrust)	Head tilt-chin lift (HCP: suspected trauma, use jaw thrust)	Head tilt-chin lift (HCP: suspected trauma, use jaw thrust)
BREATHS Initial	2 breaths at 1 second/breath	2 effective breaths at 1 second/breath	2 effective breaths at 1 second/breath
HCP: Rescue breathing without chest compression	10 to 12 breaths/min (approximately 1 breath every 5 to 6 seconds)	12 to 20 breaths/min (approximately 1 breath every 3 to 5 seconds)	12 to 20 breaths/min (approximately 1 breath every 3 to 5 seconds)
HCP: Rescue breaths for CPR with advanced airway	8 to 10 breaths/min (approximately 1 breath every 6 to 8 seconds)	8 to 10 breaths/min (approximately 1 breath every 6 to 8 seconds)	8 to 10 breaths/min (approximately 1 breath every 6 to 8 seconds)
FOREIGN-BODY AIRWAY OBSTRUCTION	Abdominal thrusts	Abdominal thrusts	Back slaps and chest thrusts
CIRCULATION HCP: Pulse check (< 10 sec)	Carotid (**HCP**: can use Femoral in a child)	Carotid (**HCP**: can use Femoral in a child)	Brachial or Femoral
COMPRESSION LANDMARKS	Center of chest, between nipples	Center of chest, between nipples	Just below nipple line
COMPRESSION METHOD Push hard and fast Allow complete recoil	**2 Hands**: Heel of 1 hand other hand on top	**2 Hands**: Heel of 1 hand with second on top or **1 Hand**: Heel of hand only	**1 rescuer**: 2 fingers **HCP**: 2 rescuers 2 thumb-encircling hands
COMPRESSION DEPTH	1 ½ inches to to 2 inches	Approximately **1/3** to ½ the depth of the chest	Approximately **1/3** to ½ the depth of the chest
COMPRESSION RATE	Approximately 100/min	Approximately 100/min	Approximately 100/min
COMPRESSION-VENTILATION-RATIO	30:2 (1 or 2 rescuers)	30:2 (single rescuer) **HCP**: 15:2 (2 rescuers)	30:2 (single rescuer) **HCP**: 15:2 (2 rescuers)
DEFIBRILLATION AED	Use adult pads. Do not use child pads/child system. **HCP**: For out-of-hospital response may provide 5 cycles/2 minutes of CPR before shock if response > 4 to 5 minutes and arrest not witnessed	**HCP**: Use AED as soon as available for sudden collapse and in-hospital. **All**: After 5 cycles of CPR (out-of-hospital). Use child pads/child system for 1 to 8 years if available. If child pads/system not available, use adult AED and pads.	No recommendation for infants <1 year of age.

*"*HCP*" designates Maneuvers used only by Healthcare providers*

Source: American Heart Association 2005. Highlights of the 2005 American Heart Association Guidelines for Cardiopulmonary Resuscitation and Emergency Cardiovascular Care. Currents, Volume 16, Number 4, Winter 2005-2006.

Automated External Defibrillator (AED)

The *American Heart Association* recommends that healthcare providers with a duty to perform CPR be trained, equipped, and authorized to perform defibrillation. In healthcare facilities, healthcare providers should be able to deliver a shock within three minutes of arrest. AED use is considered a basic life support skill.

AED: Special Situations

- **Water** Remove patient from freestanding water and dry the patient's chest before use.
- **Children** Not recommended for use in infants and children <8 years old.
- **Transdermal Medications** Do not place electrodes directly over medication patch. Remove medication patch and wipe area clean before electrode placement.
- **Implanted Pacemakers and Defibrillators (ICDs)** Place electrode pad at least 1 inch away from implanted device. If ICD is delivering shocks to victim, allow 30-60 seconds for it to complete its treatment cycle. The analysis and shock cycles of ICDs and AEDs may conflict.

AED: Operation of "Universal AED"

1. **Power On**
2. **Attach Electrode Pads** Upper-right sternal border (below clavicle) and lateral to the left nipple (a few inches below axilla).
3. **Press "Analyze" Button** If the device is equipped with an analyze button, some devices will analyze automatically. The device will analyze the cardiac rhythm (5-15 seconds). If ventricular fibrillation or a rapid ventricular tachycardia is present, an alarm or message (visual or auditory) will announce that "shock is indicated." If not, "no shock indicated" will be displayed.
4. **"Clear" Patient and Shock** Ensure everyone is "clear" (no one is in contact with patient). Press Shock button. Do not start CPR after first shock. AEDs are programmed to deliver shocks, if needed, followed by a pause. Some models do this automatically, others may require that you press Analyze after the shock.
   For the AED, rescuers should follow the directions and voice prompts of the AED they are using and should not interfere with the AED analysis as it is working.

AED and CPR

- Continue CPR until AED arrives (see page 29).
- Power "On," attach electrode pads and attempt to defibrillate (Analyze, "Clear," Shock, "Clear") up to 3 times if advised (see page 32).
- After 3 shocks or after any "no shock indicated" message, check for signs of circulation (pulse).
- If no signs of circulation, perform CPR for 1 minute.
- Check for signs of circulation and if absent continue with use of AED as prompted: Analyze, "Clear," Shock, "Clear." Repeat up to 3 shocks, then another minute of CPR if needed, etc.
- If signs of circulation are present, check breathing. If inadequate breathing: continue rescue breathing 1 breath every 5 seconds.
- If breathing is adequate, place in a recovery position and monitor.

"It may seem a strange principle to enunciate as the very first requirement in a hospital that it should do the sick no harm"
—Florence Nightingale

Notes:

Dosage Formulas

- **Amount to Administer**

(Dose ordered / Dose on hand) x Amount on hand = Amount to administer

   e.g., Order: 100mg Theophylline po q6h. Have 200mg per tablet.

$$(100/200) = 0.5 \text{ x } 1 \text{ tablet} = 0.5 \ (1/2 \text{ tablet})$$

- **Hourly Rate**

Total volume / Total # of hours infusing = Hourly rate

   e.g., Order: Infuse 1000ml NaCl over 12 hours

$$1000/12 = 83.3 \text{ ml/hr (pump rate)}$$

- **Determine Drops per Minute**

(Total volume x Drop factor) / Time in minutes = Drops per minute

  Drop Factor: Microdrip Infusion Set: 60gtt/min.

              Macrodrip Infusion Set: 15gtt/min.

If in doubt, look at the infusion set package; it will tell you the drop factor.

   e.g., Order: Infuse 1000ml NaCl over 12 hours

$$(83.3 \text{ X } 60)/60 = 83 \text{gtt/min or same order with a macrodrip}$$
$$(83.3 \text{ X } 15)/60 = 21 \text{gtt/min}$$

- **Determine Concentration**

   e.g., Order: IV fluids have 25,000 units of Heparin in 500cc of $1/2$ NS.

$$25,000 \text{u}/500 \text{cc} = 50 \text{ units/cc}$$

- **To Determine Rate for Dose per Hour**

   e.g. Order: Administer 90 mg of Theophylline per hour. The IV fluids
hanging are 1000mg of Theophylline in 250cc of D5 $1/2$ NS.

Concentration = 1000mg/250cc = 4mg/cc

Dose per hour = 90 mg per hour/4mg per cc = 22.5 cc (rate for pump)

Notes:

Locate first drug on left column. Note the appropriate number of second drug and find its location along the top row. Compatibility is found on the grid square where the name of the first drug and the number of the second drug meet

	1	2	3	4	5	6	7	8	9	10	11	12	13	14	15	16	17	18	19
Atropine (1)		C		I	C	C		C	C	C	C	C	C	C	C	C	C	C	I
Butorphanol (2) *Stadol*	C			I	I	C		C	C	C	C	C	C	C	C	C	C	C	C
Codeine (3)				I									I						
Diazepam (4) *Valium*	I	I	I		I	I		I	I	I		I	I	I	I	I	I	I	I
Fentanyl (5)	C	I		I		C		C	I	C		C	I	C	C	C	C	C	
Glycopyrrolate (6) *Robinul*	C	C		I	C			C	C	C		C	I	C	C	C	C	C	C
Heparin (7)									I		I	I							
Hydroxyzine (8) *Atarax, Vistaril*	C	C		I	C	C			C	C		C	I	C	C	C	C	C	C
Meperidine (9) *Demerol, Pethadol*	C	C		I	I	C	I	C		C		C	C	C	C	C	C	C	C
Metoclopramide (10) *Reglan,Maxolon*	C	C		I	C	C		C	C			C		C	C	C	C	C	C
Midazolam (11) *Versed*	C	C					I					C	I	C	C	C	I	C	C
Morphine (12)	C	C		I	C	C	I	C	C	C	C		I	C	C	C	C	C	C
Pentobarbital (13) *Nembutal*	C	C	I	I	I	I		I	C			I			I	I	C	I	I
Prochlorperazine (14) *Compazine*	C	C		I	C	C		C	C	C	C	C	I		C	C	C	C	C
Promethazine (15) *Phenergan*	C	C		I	C	C		C	C	C	I	C	I	C		C	C	C	C
Ranitidine (16) *Zantac*	C	C		I	C	C		C	C	C	C	C	I	C	C		C	C	C
Scopolamine Hbr (17)	C	C		I	C	C		C	C	C	I	C	C	C	C	C		I	C
Secobarbital (18)	I	I		I	I	I		I	I	I	I	I	I	I	I	I	I		I
Thiethylperazine (19) *Torecan*	C			I		C		C	C	C	C	C	I	C	C	C	C	I	

Common trade names in italics

C = Compatible

I = Incompatible

□ = No documented information

Commonly Used Analgesics in Adults

Acetaminophen (Tylenol) PO 325-650mg q4 (max 1g/qid)	**Fentanyl citrate** Preop:IM/IV 0.05-0.1mg q30-60min. Postop:IM 0.05-0.1mg q1-2hr prn
Acetaminophen & codeine PO15-60mg codeine q4 (max 360mg codeine/day)	**Ibuprofen** (Advil, Motrin, Nuprin) 200-400mg q4-6 hr (max 1,200mg/day)
Amitriptyline hydrochloride (Elavil) chronic pain PO 50-100 mg/day	**Meperidine HCL** (Demerol) PO/IM/SC 50-100 mgq3-4hr, continuous IV: 15-35mg/hr
Acetaminophen & hydrocodone (Lorcet 10/650) PO 1 tabs q4-6hr (max 6 tabs/24hr)	**Morphine** IM/SC 10-20mg/70kg q4h. IV 2.5-15mg/70kg in 4-5ml H20 over 4-5min
Aspirin PO 325-600mg q4	Naproxen (Naprosyn) mild to moderate pain, initial 550mg then 275mg q6-8hr prn (max 1,375mg/day)
Codeine sulfate PO/IV/IM, SC 15-60mg q4-6hr (max 360mg/qd)	Oxycodone HCL (OxyContin, Roxicodone) PO 10-30mg q4hr individualized dose

Insulin Preparations

Type of Insulin	Time of onset (hr)	Peak of action (hr)	Duration of action (hr)	Appearance
Rapid acting				
Lispro (Humalog)	15 min	40-60 min	46 min half-life	Clear
Regular	<1	2-4	4-6	Clear
Crystalline zinc	<1	2-4	5-8	Clear
Semilente	1-2	3-10	10-16	Cloudy
Intermediate				
NPH	1-2	4-12	18-24	Cloudy
Globin zinc	2-4	6-10	12-18	Clear
Lente	1-3	6-15	18-24	Cloudy
Slow acting				
Protamine zinc	4-8	14-24	36+	Cloudy
Ultralente	4-8	10-30	28-36	Cloudy

*Consult a drug reference guide for further specific information including contraindications, interactions and other nursing clinical concerns.

NANDA Nursing Diagnoses*

*By permission, *Nursing Diagnoses: Definitions & Classification* 2001–2002 NANDA

• **Exchanging**	**(Exchanging cont.)**
Imbalanced nutrition: More than body requirements	Risk for fluid volume imbalance
Imbalanced nutrition: Less than body requirements	Excess fluid volume
	Deficient fluid volume
Risk for imbalanced nutrition: More than body requirements	Risk for deficient fluid volume
	Decreased cardiac output
Risk for infection	Impaired gas exchange
Risk for imbalanced body temperature	Ineffective airway clearance
	Ineffective breathing pattern
Hypothermia	Impaired spontaneous ventilation
Hyperthermia	Dysfunctional ventilatory weaning response
Ineffective thermoregulation	
Autonomic dysreflexia	Risk for injury
Risk for autonomic dysreflexia	Risk for suffocation
Constipation	Risk for poisoning
Perceived constipation	Risk for trauma
Diarrhea	Risk for aspiration
Bowel incontinence	Risk for disuse syndrome
Risk for constipation	Latex allergy response
Impaired urinary elimination	Risk for latex allergy response
Stress urinary incontinence	Ineffective protection
Reflex urinary incontinence	Impaired tissue integrity
Urge urinary incontinence	Impaired oral mucous membrane
Functional urinary incontinence	Impaired skin integrity
Total urinary incontinence	Risk for impaired skin integrity
Risk for urge urinary incontinence	Impaired dentition
Urinary retention	Decreased intracranial adaptive capacity
Ineffective tissue perfusion (specify type: renal, cerebral, cardiopulmonary, gastrointestinal, peripheral)	Disturbed energy field
	• **Communicating**
	Impaired verbal communication

NANDA Nursing Diagnoses (cont.)

• **Relating**
Impaired social interaction
Social isolation
Risk for loneliness
Ineffective role performance
Deficient parenting
Risk for deficient parenting
Risk for impaired parent/infant/child attachment
Sexual dysfunction
Interrupted family processes
Caregiver role strain
Risk for caregiver role strain
Altered family processes: Alcoholism
Parental role conflict
Ineffective sexuality patterns

• **Valuing**
Spiritual distress
Risk for spiritual distress
Readiness for enhanced spiritual well-being

• **Choosing**
Ineffective coping
Impaired adjustment
Defensive coping
Ineffective denial
Disabled family coping
Compromised family coping
Readiness for enhanced family coping
Readiness for enhanced community coping

(**Choosing** cont.)
Ineffective community coping
Ineffective therapeutic regimen management
Noncompliance (specify)
Ineffective family therapeutic regimen management
Ineffective community therapeutic regimen management
Effective therapeutic regimen management
Decisional conflict (specify)
Health-seeking behaviors (specify)

• **Moving**
Impaired physical mobility
Risk for peripheral neurovascular dysfunction
Risk for perioperative-positioning injury
Impaired walking
Impaired wheelchair mobility
Impaired transfer ability
Impaired bed mobility
Activity intolerance
Fatigue
Risk for activity intolerance
Sleep pattern disturbance
Sleep deprivation
Deficient diversional activity
Impaired home maintenance
Ineffective health maintenance
Delayed surgical recovery
Adult failure to thrive

NANDA Nursing Diagnoses (cont.)

(Moving cont.)
Feeding self-care deficit
Impaired swallowing
Ineffective breastfeeding
Interrupted breastfeeding
Effective breastfeeding
Ineffective infant feeding pattern
Bathing/hygiene self-care deficit
Dressing/grooming self-care deficit
Toileting self-care deficit
Delayed growth and development
Risk for delayed development
Risk for disproportionate growth
Relocation stress syndrome
Risk for disorganized infant behavior
Disorganized infant behavior
Readiness for enhanced organized
  infant behavior

• **Perceiving**
Disturbed body image
Disturbed self-esteem
Chronic low self-esteem
Situational low self-esteem
Disturbed personal identity
Disturbed sensory perception
  (specify: visual, auditory, gustatory,
  tactile, olfactory, kinesthetic)
Unilateral neglect
Hopelessness
Powerlessness

• **Knowing**
Deficient knowledge (specify)
Impaired environmental
  interpretation syndrome

(Knowing cont.)
Acute confusion
Chronic confusion
Disturbed thought processes
Impaired memory

• **Feeling**
Acute pain
Chronic pain
Nausea
Dysfunctional grieving
Anticipatory grieving
Chronic sorrow
Risk for other-directed violence
Risk for self-mutilation
Risk for self-directed violence
Post-trauma syndrome
Rape-trauma syndrome
Rape-trauma syndrome:
  Compound reaction
Rape-trauma syndrome:
  Silent reaction
Risk for post-trauma syndrome
Anxiety
Death anxiety
Fear

• **New Nursing Dx, April 2000**
Risk for relocation stress syndrome
Risk for suicide
Self-mutilation
Risk for powerlessness
Risk for situational low self-esteem
Wandering
Risk for falls

Web Sites

- *www.americanheart.org*   American Heart Association

- *www.stroke.org*   National Stroke Association

- *www.medlineplus.gov*   Health information provided by the U.S. National Library of Medicine and the National Institutes of Health

- *www.diabetes.org*   American Diabetes Association

- *www.hfsa.org*   Heart Failure Society of America

- *www.nhlbi.nih.gov/guidelines*   National Heart, Lung, and Blood Institute

- *www.aidsinfo.nih.gov*   HIV infection clinical guidelines. A service of the U.S. Department of Health and Human Services

- *www.cdc.gov*   Centers for Disease Control

- *www.fda.gov*   Food and Drug Administration

References

Alspach, J. (Ed.) (2005). *Core Curriculum for Critical Care Nursing* (6th ed.). Philadelphia, PA: Saunders.

American Diabetes Association (2005). "Summary of Revisions for the 2005 Clinical Practice Recommendations." *Diabetes Care* 28, S3.

American Heart Association (2005). *2005 Guidelines for CPR and ECC.* Dallas, TX: American Heart Association.

American Heart Association (2005). *Heart Disease and Stroke Statistics* (2005 update). Dallas, Texas: American Heart Association.

Anderson N. K. (Ed.) (2002). *Mosby's Medical, Nursing & Allied Health Dictionary* (6th ed.). Philadelphia, PA: WB Saunders.

Cannon, C.P., Braunwald, E., McCabe, C.H., et al. (2004). "Intensive versus moderate lipid lowering with statins after acute coronary syndromes." *New England Journal of Medicine* 350, no. 15: 1495-1504.

Desai, S. (2004) *Clinician's Guide to Laboratory Medicine* (3rd ed.). Hudson, OH: Lexi-Comp, Inc.

Ferri, F. (2004). *A Practical Guide to Clinical Laboratory Medicine and Diagnostic Imaging*. Philadelphia, PA: Mosby.

Freedberg, I., Eisen, A., Wolff, K., et al. (2003). *Fitzpatrick's Dermatology in General Medicine* (6th ed.). New York: McGraw-Hill.

Hankins J. et al. (2001). *Infusion Therapy in Clinical Practice.* Philadelphia, PA: WB Saunders.

References (cont.)

Jarvis, C. (2003). *Physical Examination and Health Assessment* (4th ed.). Philadelphia, PA: WB Saunders.

LeFever, J. K. (2004). *Laboratory and Diagnostic Tests with Nursing Implications.* (7th ed.). Upper Saddle River, NJ: Prentice Hall.

National Heart, Lung, and Blood Institute (2001). *Third Report of the National Cholesterol Education Program.* (Publication No. 01-3670). Bethesda, MD: National Institutes of Health.

North American Nursing Diagnosis Association (2001). *NANDA Nursing Diagnosis: Definitions and Classifications 2000-2002.* Philadelphia, PA: NANDA.

Rasmusson, K.D., Hall, J.A., Vesty, J.C., et al. (2006). "Managing the heart failure epidemic: The evolving role of nurse specialists." *Topics in Advanced Practice Nursing eJournal* 5, no. 4. Accessed 1/10/2006 from *www.medscape.com/viewarticle/518386.*

Spratto, G. & Woods, A. (2006). *2007 PDR Nurse's Drug Handbook.* Clifton Park, NY: Delmar Learning.

Swartz, H. M. (2005). *Textbook of Physical Diagnosis: History and Examination* (5th ed.). Philadelphia, PA: WB Saunders.

Urden, D. L. et al. (2005). *Thelan's Critical Care nursing: Diagnosis and Management* (5th ed.). St. Louis, MO: Mosby.

U.S. Public Health Service (2001). *Updated Guidelines for the Management of Occupational Exposures to HBV, HCV, and HIV and Recommendations for Postexposure Prophylaxis.* Washington, DC: U.S. Public Health Service.